T. Lee Baumann, M.D.

Clearing the Air: Art of the Bowel Movement
by
T. Lee Baumann, M.D.

Revised Printing: March 2015

Printed in the U.S.A.
CreateSpace
7290-B Investment Drive
North Charleston, SC 29418, USA

Baumann, T. Lee, 1950-
    Clearing the Air: Art of the Bowel Movement
    / by T. Lee Baumann

Includes endnotes and index.
    ISBN: 1490381252
    ISBN-13: 978-1490381251

This book is dedicated to the world's burgeoning population of the elderly, including this author.

Also by
T. LEE BAUMANN:

God at the Speed of Light

Window to God

The Akashic Light

The Seagull Project (fiction)

Matter to Mind to Consciousness

Nondenominational Quantum Spirituality Lay Manual for Hospice Patients and Their Families

The Dark Conscious (fiction)

Sin Denominación Espiritualidad Cuántica Manual Laico para Pacientes de Hospicio y sus Familias

Medusa of Time

Table of Contents:

Foreword

In 1994, I was shown a copy of a funny book, at least for most Americans. It was entitled *The Gas We Pass: The Story of Farts* by Shinta Cho,[1] first published in Japan in 1978.

As a physician, I immediately thought that this was a "gag" book, published purely as an entertainment vehicle. Certainly, as Americans, the fart is a formidable topic of comedy, relished and utilized to its full extent by most comics at some point in their comedy routines.

I was soon enlightened, however, that this was a serious topic in Japan, and this book existed as a classic in Japan to edify children on the subject of flatus and its associated subject: the bowel movement.

I practiced medicine in the 1970's and 80's. This was a time when researchers were just beginning to learn the power, positive effects, and necessity of dietary fiber. Prior to this era, most of the general public considered fiber as purely an unnecessary constituent of many foods: an ingredient that could not be absorbed and was of no medicinal or medical value.

How times have changed. We now appreciate dietary fiber as a necessary part of any healthy diet and one of the major ingredients for maintaining digestive health and normal intestinal activity.

With the general age of the world's vast population increasing at an explosive rate, we rely more and more on the reliable bowel movement to maintain our psychological health and feeling of physical wellness.

There are many variables involved in the human bowel movement, not the least of which is the gastrocolic reflex—meaning that each time food enters the stomach, the colon is set into action. Utilizing this sole example alone, it is easy to see that the modern worker cannot afford the luxury of running to the restroom after every meal—though our evolutionary history would encourage us do just that.

Indeed, with a little education and simple modification to the diet, we can turn a grumpy and retentive bowel into a happy one. I was approaching the age of 60 when I had my first colonoscopy. It was completely and 100% normal because of my 30+ years of fiber supplementation. Let's face it, we all know that a healthy and "regular" old person (that includes this author) means a happier elder and immediate family and/or caretaker.

SPECIAL NOTE AND DISCLAIMER: The reader should always speak to his/her family physician before implementing any recommendation as set forth within the pages of this book. Even seemingly benign suggestions may have dire consequences under the right circumstances, so caution and prevention are always advised.

Chapter 1: The Digestive System—Why We Eat

The number of calories that our bodies require depends primarily upon our height, age, and level of physical activity. A tall, young athlete requires substantially more calories than a short, sedentary, older person. One additional determining factor is the higher metabolic rate of a younger person. These differences explain in large part why, at age fifty, we find ourselves eating less but packing on the pounds.

The digestive process begins in the mouth, where our teeth grind and shred our food. Saliva mixes with the food to ease swallowing. Saliva contains the first digestive enzyme, salivary amylase, which begins to break down large carbohydrate molecules. Researchers estimate that our bodies secrete a total of 1 to 1.5 liters of saliva per day.

From the time that the initial food bolus passes down the esophagus and hits the stomach, a coating of protective mucus serves to safeguard the lining of the stomach from the potent digestive enzymes and hydrochloric acid that are released here. Hence, alcohol, drugs, and any disease processes which affect this protective layer of mucus will leave the stomach, adjoining esophagus, and proximal intestine vulnerable to erosion and ulceration.

When the digested contents of the stomach (chyme) pass into the small intestine, the main work of nutrient absorption begins. Digestive enzymes from the liver, pancreas, and intestinal wall all aid in breaking down the chyme further for eventual absorption into the bloodstream. Ninety-five (95) percent of all of our ingested nutrients are absorbed in the small intestine. The small intestine is approximately 7 meters (23 feet) in length. The large surface area of this organ enables it to perform its absorptive function as well as it does.

Following the absorption of most nutrients, the remaining contents pass into the large intestine or colon. Although the most recognized function of the colon is water reabsorption, the contents also undergo fermentation by the bacteria present here, allowing even more nutrients to become available for absorption. It is this process of colonic fermentation which is largely responsible for flatus production.

Since flatus exists as such a popular topic of conversation in our mundane human existence, I will offer the following research statistics:

1. The malodor of most farts derives from the sulfur content of our ingested foods. Hence, pinto beans are a major offender.
2. The human body produces between 500 and 1500 cc of flatus per day.
3. The volume of a single flatulence event can vary widely, and articles claim averages (depending on the study group) for everything from just a few cc's to nearly 400 cc per event.

4. The first flatulence upon awaking in the morning is generally the largest, conceivably from accumulation of gas during the night.

5. The intestines are directly responsible for around 75% of the volume of flatus produced, with hydrogen, carbon dioxide, and methane being the main constituents.

6. The news media have recently communicated the prominent contribution of livestock to the planet's greenhouse gas problem. While cattle contribute to about twenty percent of the world's methane emissions, only 5-10% of this methane comes from their flatus. The vast majority of their methane production comes from exhaling and belching!

7. Intestinal gases, including ingested gas from eating and swallowing, can progress through the entire digestive tract at rates far surpassing those of their liquid and solid counterparts. These gases also pass through the intestinal tract more efficiently in the

upright than horizontal position.

8. The wide variability of sounds emitted with flatulence are dependent upon the size, shape, and position of the rectum and anus, as well as the tightness of the anal sphincter and the velocity of the expelled gas.

9. Depending upon the culture, audible flatulence may be received with embarrassment, humor, or indifference.

Once the contents of the bowels reach the final segment of the large bowel, the rectum, the process of digestion is essentially complete. From this point onward, the process transitions from one of digestion to evacuation.

Chapter 2: Evolution, History, and the Importance of Fiber
God helps those who are willing to help themselves.

When the products of digestion finally reach the rectum, the only obstacle remaining to prevent a socially-embarrassing evacuation is the anal sphincter. As the rectum fills with fecal contents, stretch receptors prompt the rectal muscles into action, and the urge to defecate results.

In general however, the anus will heed the call and thwart the rectum from inducing any untoward events. Indeed, the anus is a miraculous organ that has the rare capacity to differentiate between the presence of solid, liquid, or gas and, in most cases, successfully retain or expel them individually and on an as-needed basis. Consider that this venerable product of evolution, one which receives less than its fair share of deserved respect, is all that separates us from social banishment.

Unfortunately for us, if the rectal impulse to defecate is delayed by the anus over a prolonged period (any duration is too long as far as the rectum is concerned), the rectum will retire the bolus of material back to the sigmoid colon. Think of the rectum as a long balloon partially filled (or pressurized) with air. Consider what happens if extra pressure is applied to the balloon and its contents—that is, you squeeze the balloon. If one end of the balloon is blocked (i.e., tied off, representing the constricted anus), the pressurized contents (the air in the balloon) will seek out the path of least resistance (the other, under-inflated end of the balloon, representing the sigmoid colon). If the anal sphincter has constricted and refuses passage of the rectal contents to the outside, the contracting rectum will propel the bolus back to the sigmoid colon as the latter eventually relaxes against the superior strength of its clinched anal opponent.

With the fecal contents now back in the

colon, the rectal contractions and urge to defecate dissipate. Here the colon will aptly respond again to its assigned duty of water reabsorption, and it does this job well. The bolus will lose its previous natural pliability and begin to harden. Think of thick mud hardening into bricks. It's much the same with the colon, and constipation will result.

Yet, the veritable ring of anal musculature which has caused all this trouble, and on which so much depends (pun intended), is one of the most neglected anatomical parts of the entire human body. The disrespect that it endures is legendary.

Most humans go to all extremes to avoid any type of direct contact with this forbidden area. Following a bowel movement, many cultures utilize bidets or washlets so as to limit the amount of necessary contact.

In cultures such as America where bidets and washlets are not the norm, any direct contact that may be required always includes separation of the hand or fingers by intervening squares of tissue or a sacrificial washcloth. Soiled tissues are quickly disposed of with a simple flick of the toilet handle.

A sullied washcloth, on the other hand, is gingerly lifted with the thumb and forefinger by one uncontaminated corner and placed quickly into the next day's load of laundry. All unnecessary eye contact with the tainted fabric is also to be avoided.

In some individuals, the anus doesn't even receive this degree of inattention and is *totally* disregarded. In these rare circumstances, the importance of clean and preferably fresh underwear becomes paramount.

We must commend evolution for its underappreciated success of the anus. Yet, both the anus and rectum require our undivided attention in achieving ultimate success in its intended civil duties.

As both owner and master over these two organs, we are expected to exercise a certain degree of discipline and restraint to allow for our continued participation within the social community. Not only is this degree of self-control expected, it is mandatory.

On the other hand, overzealous retention of our rectal contents can lead to an equally uncomfortable situation: constipation or impaction. This predicament is to be avoided when possible. Thus, we are constantly confronted with maintaining the delicate balance between spontaneous elimination at one end and fecal impaction on the other.

There are several excellent ways to enable us to walk this fine line.

Our ancestors, by necessity, ingested a significantly greater percentage of fiber than our refined food offer today. As such, our bowels evolved with fiber as a prominent constituent of the normal diet. With fiber, our ancestors were "regular," and *constipation* was not in the Old World lexicon. The problem just didn't exist.

In contrast, the modern diet sorely lacks fiber. Researchers estimate that people living in developed countries ingest only between 20-50% of the daily recommended intake of fiber.

Constipation is a now a common malady of developed countries, and the explosive use of laxatives has created its own host of health issues. Not only do many laxatives have unpleasant side effects (to be discussed), but some have significant risks with long-term use and can cause long-standing physical pathology.

The prevalence of constipation in North America is far from consistent—with ranges extending from 1.9 to 27.2% (most estimates are 12-19%), and females outnumber males 2.2 to 1.[2]

Constipation is a symptom—not a disease. Hence, chronic sufferers of constipation should seek medical help to exclude other causes such as hypothyroidism, colorectal cancer, and the effects of medications to name a few.

The Rome II Criteria[3] for constipation require two or more of the following symptoms:

1. Straining during at least 25% of defecations
2. Lumpy or hard stools in at least 25% of defecations
3. Sensation of incomplete evacuation for at least 25% of defecations
4. Sensation of anorectal

obstruction/blockage for at least 25% of defecations

5. Manual maneuvers [used] to facilitate at least 25% of defecations (e.g., digital evacuation, support of the pelvic floor)
6. Fewer than three defecations per week
7. Loose stools are rarely present without the use of laxatives
8. Insufficient criteria for irritable bowel syndrome

[The above] Criteria fulfilled for the last 3 months with symptom onset at least 6 months prior to diagnosis.

For many if not most of us, our diet is the main cause of constipation. Depending on the source, the lack of adequate dietary fiber and inadequate hydration vie for the number one and two reasons for this modern malady.

To help emphasize the need for proper hydration, I must point out that my own experiences with constipation, despite the 40+ grams of fiber that I consume every day, stem from instances where I do not adequately hydrate for periods ranging between 4-6 hours. Usually, this is simply because I become preoccupied in some work project, and my bowels pay the price. The colon is extremely efficient at scavenging fluid from its lumenal contents when required to maintain bodily hydration—whether fiber is present in the bowel or not.

Yet, with adequate liquids, fiber assists our bowels at working most efficiently. The lack of fiber is a major cause, not only for constipation, but also for another common bowel ailment known as diverticulosis, included within the spectrum of diverticular diseases. Diverticulosis is an *asymptomatic* process whereby outpouchings of the lining of the colon occur through its muscular layer. This pathology results from the increased intra-colonic pressures generated by the act of "bearing down" to evacuate the rectum. Think of your bowel wall as a rubber balloon. Blow hard enough, and it will inflate and expand. If you generate enough pressure, the bowel wall may push through its outer muscular layer and form a small secondary "balloon" peeking out through the other side. These outpouchings would not be of any concern except that they can become infected (diverticulitis[4]), bleed, or even perforate (the balloon "pops")—all potentially life-threatening conditions.

From our modern day eradication of natural fiber from the diet, the incidence of diverticulosis has become so prevalent that, in developed countries, 50% of people over the age of 60 have the disease.

A *low* fiber diet concomitant with recurrent constipation and the use of stimulant laxatives further increases the risk for bleeding and infection in diverticulosis patients.

The best way to avoid all of the above (that is, constipation, the need for laxatives, and the development of diverticulosis and its complications) is to simply increase your intake of dietary fiber (and the associated fluids they require). This task is not as easy as it might sound in light of the ubiquitous presence of "refined" grains in most of the current foods found on our grocery store shelves. Thus, in my estimation, the only *practical* way to increase our daily intake of fiber, short of becoming a rabbit, is to buy fiber additives to supplement our diet.

Supplementing our diet with fiber is fraught with its own risks. Depending on the health resource, medical association, and your sex and age, the recommended daily intake of fiber may range anywhere from 20 to 40 grams per day. The best recommendation,[5] I believe, comes from the Institute of Medicine which recommends 14 grams for every 1000 calories consumed.[6]

I cannot overemphasize that any intake of fiber requires an adequate intake of fluid. Not only do dietary fibers require sufficient liquids to perform their health functions (and also to avoid their complications), but dehydration alone is a common cause of constipation.

History of Fiber

I used to pride myself in the 1980's for the moniker I received from my grateful patients. They called me "Dr. Fiber." Thus, it was with some surprise that I read that I had been beaten in the use of this endearing term by one of my medical peers just a few years earlier. This physician, known as "the fiber man," was Dr. Denis P. Burkitt, the same surgeon who garnered fame for his groundbreaking research on a childhood cancer which would bear his name: Burkitt's lymphoma.

Dr. Burkitt made a second discovery, however—one that forms the topic of this discussion. He observed from work in Africa that many diseases prevalent in our Western culture (heart disease, obesity, and certain cancers and gastrointestinal ailments) were almost nonexistent in Africa. He concluded that a cause-and-effect relationship existed as a result of dietary fiber. His book, *Don't Forget Fibre in your Diet*,[7] was an international best seller in 1979, the year I graduated from my medical residency. Dr. Burkitt recognized that the colonic bacteria differed significantly between his African and Western study groups, with the African subjects possessing a much higher proportion of *Streptococci*. In addition, the

African group had a higher percentage of neutral (compared to acidic) steroids in their colons. Dr. Burkitt correctly hypothesized that the deleterious effects of potential carcinogens within the bowel would be lessened by a more rapid transit through the bowel (with decreased exposure time within the gut), plus incurring the beneficial effects of the healthier colonic environment. History, as it turned out, would support Dr. Burkitt's theory.

There are a wide variety of fibers—each with its own special characteristics that may be successfully utilized, depending upon one's own physical and social needs and idiosyncrasies.

There are two primary types of beneficial fiber. *Soluble* fiber indicates a fiber that is soluble (dissolves) in water and typically slows bowel motility, including gastric emptying. *Insoluble* fiber, on the other hand, is *not* soluble in water and typically speeds bowel motility.

Popular forms of soluble fiber include psyllium seed husk (Metamucil) and the beta-glucans such as oat bran and barley.

Other types of soluble fiber may be found naturally in pectin, fruits, dried beans, and peas. Soluble fiber absorbs water, forming a gelatinous compound in the process. Concomitant fluids are required to keep the mixture fluid.

Physicians will often employ soluble fibers for gastrointestinal disorders that have elements of diarrhea[8] or even components of both diarrhea and constipation (such as irritable bowel syndrome[9]).

Soluble fibers are more likely to ferment during their passage through the bowel and produce gas, but both soluble and insoluble fibers are capable of fermentation.

Some soluble fibers also produce metabolic byproducts with beneficial anti-inflammatory effects that may alleviate some forms of inflammatory bowel disease (e.g., Crohn's disease, ulcerative colitis, and some forms of antibiotic-induced diarrhea).

Several recent studies even reveal that certain fibers suppress appetite through mechanisms other than just increasing the sensation of fullness:

1. [M]any foods high in fermentable fiber, such as cabbage, beans and most sweet fruit and vegetables, are unable to be digested by the intestine directly.

Instead, intestinal bacteria ferments these fibers into short-chain fatty acids, including butyrate and propionate. These fatty acids can then be absorbed by the body...

These findings suggest that it is the glucose-producing activity of the intestines as a result of propionate and butyrate, and intestinal bacteria, that cause fermentable fibers to protect against obesity and diabetes.[10]

2. In mammals—both rodents and humans—fiber is digested by bacteria in the colon, which release various chemicals as they work. Fiber gets broken down into acetate, among other things.

In one set of experiments, the researchers fed a group of mice a diet that was high in a type of fiber called inulin (not to be confused with the hormone insulin), which is found in foods such as bananas and garlic. Another group of mice was fed a diet low in that type of fiber.

After two months, the mice with the high-inulin diet had gained less weight, and an analysis of their colon content showed more acetate compared with the mice on the low-inulin diet.

[The article wisely points out that you cannot achieve the same results by merely drinking vinegar, as most of the acetic acid is digested in the proximal gut and broken down.][11]

3. Bell and his colleagues…fed mice fibre labelled with carbon-13…The fibre was fermented as usual into acetate, which turned up not only in the gut, but also in the hypothalamus, a part of the brain known to be involved in regulating appetite. There, the researchers found, it was metabolized through the glutamine-glutamate cycle, which is involved in controlling the release of neurotransmitters associated with appetite control.[12]

Hence, the evidence for fiber in the successful treatment over obesity is ever growing.

Soluble fibers additionally lower harmful cholesterol by binding bile acids (made up of cholesterol) in the small intestine and hinder the bile acids' subsequent reabsorption into the bloodstream. Similarly, some types of soluble fiber lessen sugar absorption and provide a useful adjunct in the treatment of diabetes.

My favorite soluble fiber is psyllium. It is economical, highly effective as a soluble fiber, and practical. Psyllium is derived from the plant *Plantago psyllium*, but the husk and seed of *Plantago ovata* is also commonly referred to as psyllium. The standard form of psyllium sold in the stores is obtained by milling the seed of *P. ovata* to remove the hulls. The predominant active ingredient of psyllium husk is hemicellulose. The whole seed consists of a variety of 65% soluble and 35% insoluble polysaccharides (including cellulose, hemicellulose, and lignin). The natural psyllium seed's ability to form a gel in water has evolved as a strategic evolutionary advantage, allowing the seeds to retain needed moisture for survival.

Insoluble fibers have their own special set of properties and benefits. These fibers consist of the structural elements of plant cell walls. They are found in the peels of fruit, the husks of grains, and in legumes. The whole grain fibers include wheat and corn bran, and the legumes include beans and peas. Grain fibers act as natural laxatives that increase the transit of foods through the entire intestine. None of these insoluble fibers mix or dissolve in water— nor are they digestible.

Wheat bran is easily obtainable in products such as Kellogg's All Bran cereal.[13] This convenient fiber product contains the non-digestible portions of the wheat grain. I recommend this insoluble form of wheat bran for its bulking properties. Bulk fibers aid the body in two ways. They help to induce a feeling of fullness and satiation by merely stretching the lumens of the stomach and intestine, and they are the best fibers for treating constipation and preventing the development of diverticulosis.

Another wheat product known as Benefiber is a wheat dextrin and is a *soluble* fiber. It should not be confused as an insoluble fiber.

Unfortunately, despite all the positive reasons for taking fiber, there are always verbal excuses for *not* taking it. Following are several arguments that I often hear for not taking fiber:

1. "Fiber tastes awful."
2. "Fiber gives me diarrhea."
3. "Fiber gives me gas. I feel bloated all the time."
4. "It's impossible to eat *that* much fiber."
5. "I already have diverticular disease. It's too late to help me."
6. "I never get constipated, so I don't need fiber."

I do not accept any of the above excuses. All fibers exude some benefit, and there are compelling ways to overcome complaints such as the flat taste, the gastrointestinal problems (many of which are associated with a bowel that is unaccustomed to a "normal" fiber load),[14] and the presence of already-existent diverticular disease.

The majority of medical studies have documented the many health benefits of dietary fiber. However, like anything else in the field of medicine, there exist the typical phases of acceptance: discovery, acceptance, then skepticism, and lastly either final acceptance or rejection.

Coffee is one of many classic such examples.[15] Its first recorded use dates back to the 15th century. It gained historical popularity as a safe mental stimulant and even touted as a "miracle drug." After centuries of proven efficacy and relative safety, it eventually became maligned as a complex and even dangerous drug with a bevy of adverse effects. These risks included gastritis, ulcers, insomnia, anxiety, high blood pressure, heart disease (conflicting results), glaucoma, high cholesterol (from unfiltered coffee[16]), and various drug interactions.

In recent years, however, coffee has undergone a resurgence in popularity, largely due to research which has demonstrated a host of beneficial effects unrelated to coffee's caffeine content. These studies have revealed that moderate coffee consumption (3-6 cups/day) may reduce one's general over-all mortality (women more so than men). Decaffeinated coffee appears to offer the same benefits as its caffeinated counterpart. Specific alleged benefits include reduced risks for such diverse diseases as Alzheimer's, gallstones, Parkinson's, diabetes, hepatic cirrhosis, hepatocellular carcinoma, a host of other cancers (oral, pharyngeal, esophageal, breast, endometrial, and prostate), cardiovascular disease, constipation, dental caries, high blood pressure, and even gout (men only). Far from being a wonder drug, however, such benefits should always be interpreted cautiously. The benefits were associated only with moderate coffee consumption and for patients in whom the stimulant effects would not pose a medical risk.

Of course, I would be remiss in this text not to emphasize coffee's efficient stimulant effects upon bowel motility.

Combine coffee with the neurologically-induced gastrocolic reflex of any meal, and you have a meaningful trigger to call many bowels into action. After the typical overnight fast following sleep, this potent combination of colonic stimulants upon the still-sleepy bowel is especially efficacious—one to which nearly every morning coffee drinker can attest.

A few stray fragments of the medical community are still hovering between the phases of skepticism and final acceptance as it pertains to dietary fiber and the prevention of diverticulosis. At least one recent study is refuting much of the past research that appeared to establish a clear link between fiber and the prevention of diverticular disease. There may well be additional such studies to surface, but I predict the majority of these studies will corroborate fiber's past beneficial links. Similar to the rare research study that goes against the grain of proven historical data, I suspect that flaws in study design or other inadvertent errors will explain these contradictory results.

Differences in medical studies and their

outcomes can depend upon a wide variety of factors that may unintentionally influence the results. Such unpredictable variables include but not limited to the following:

1. Study size (Smaller studies are less representative of the general public than larger studies.)
2. Age, sex, and medical conditions of the subjects
3. Degree of compliance of the subjects (did they really consume the fiber as directed?)
4. Type of fiber utilized in the study, including the brand, the type of manufacturing process involved, and whether the fiber was soluble or insoluble
5. Amounts of fluid consumed in conjunction with the fiber (Constipation and other problems may occur with insufficient fluid intake.)
6. Other ill-defined contributing variables as diverse as the effects of medications or ingested irritants on

the bowel and other factors including undiagnosed disease states and infectious agents

Certainly, most past medical studies indicate a preponderance of beneficial effects from dietary fiber. These include reported reductions in the incidence or complications of some the following conditions:

1. Breast cancer (soluble fiber)
2. Ovarian cancer (soluble fiber)
3. Bowel cancer (both soluble and insoluble fibers)
4. Chronic inflammatory bowel diseases (fermentable soluble fibers)
5. Irritable bowel syndrome (soluble fiber)
6. Coronary heart disease (soluble fiber)
7. High blood glucose in pre-diabetics and diabetics (soluble fibers predominantly, but insoluble fibers also play a role)
8. High cholesterol (soluble fiber)
9. Obesity (both soluble and insoluble fibers may add to the feeling of

satiety)

10. Constipation (insoluble fibers predominantly, but soluble fibers also play a role)

11. Hemorrhoids (insoluble fibers predominantly, but soluble fibers also play a role)

12. Diverticulosis (predominately insoluble fiber)

13. Complications of already-established diverticular disease, e.g., infection and perforation (predominately insoluble fibers for prevention—with caveats to be discussed)

The most controversial issue relative to fiber, which I believe has divided the most physicians, is whether a patient who has recovered from an episode of diverticulitis should now engage in a high fiber or a low fiber (low "residue") diet. How the medical community can be so diametrically opposed boils down to training—a hard paradigm to break in medicine. Yet, that is the state of the art in the medical field—and is certainly witnessed in other vocations as well. One physician will recommend one treatment. Another physician will recommend the exact opposite. This is why patients should always get second or third opinions when in doubt regarding either diagnosis or treatment.

To me and a growing number of physicians, the preponderance of evidence appears to successfully argue that a high fiber diet, especially one high in insoluble fiber (e.g., wheat bran), lessens the incidence of high intra-colonic pressures and, hence, worsening of patients' diverticuloses and the potential risk of perforation.

On the other side of the coin, many currently practicing physicians believe that the ingestion of any nonabsorbable material (i.e., any type of fiber—soluble or insoluble) predisposes existing diverticula to the risk of infection or bleeding. These doctors recommend a low residue diet, with a total abstinence of the likes of nuts, seeds, corn, and popcorn to fend off recurrences of diverticulitis. They have fully rejected the use of fiber for this ailment. In my experience, this is an outdated but not uncommon practice. There is no evidence that these foods increase the risk for diverticulitis. In fact, the opposite is more likely: such high fiber foods may well protect against such a recurrence.[17]

Then there are those physicians who stand somewhere in the middle. These are doctors who ask their patients to avoid insoluble fibers and bulking agents (including nuts and seeds) but allow or even recommend the use of soluble fibers. These practitioners are solidly fixed between the skepticism and acceptance phases—not having yet made up their minds.

Most all physicians *do* agree that during the *acute* treatment phase of diverticulitis, while the infection and inflammation are still active, that all forms of fiber (and many foods) should be avoided. The purpose of this is to place the bowel "at rest" (as much as that is possible) to allow and promote healing of the diseased bowel. Once the bowel has rested, recovered, and is free of symptoms, however, many (but still not all) leading institutions recommend a gradual increase in fiber to the recommended allotments (depending upon the reference source and the patient's sex and age). These institutions include the likes of Stanford,[18] University of Maryland Medical Center,[19] the University of California at San Francisco (UCSF),[20] the National Digestive Diseases Information Clearinghouse (NDDIC),[21] and the Cleveland Clinic[22] just to name a few.

As with so much in medicine, even these physicians and medical institutions can't totally agree on the few things that they do agree on. Confusing? Of course. For instance, many institutions recommend that patients gradually resume high fiber diets following an episode of diverticulitis, but they can't agree on the timing. Stanford recommends adding fiber once "your flares subside." UCSF recommends reinstituting fiber 2-4 days and the NDDIC "a few days" after symptoms have eased. The Cleveland Clinic, however, conservatively recommends resuming fiber a "month or so after the infection resolves."

As noted earlier, I support the Institute of Medicine's uncomplicated dosage recommendation of 14 grams of fiber for every 1000 calories consumed,[23] and this would pertain for fiber goals following an episode of diverticulitis as well. This counsel's recommendation obviates the need for separating fiber intake based upon age and sex.

There is little risk of overindulging on fiber, but some risks do exist. The potential complications may include undue flatulence (mainly the soluble fibers) and, more importantly, decreased absorption of some medications and nutrients. This diminished absorption can result from any combination of binding of digestive bile acids by soluble fibers as well as the decreased transit time through the intestine incurred by mainly insoluble fibers. Because of these potential actions of fiber upon drug absorption, most physicians recommend that oral medications be taken at least 1 hour *before* or 2 - 4 hours *after* taking fiber,[24] but, as always, check with your physician.

Aside from fiber's infrequent but potential interactions with some medications, fiber also has some positive interactions. One of these involves the cholesterol-lowering agents known as bile acid sequestrants (including the medications, colestipol and cholestyramine). These drugs act through the binding of bile acids (an effect also of some soluble fibers) secreted in the process of digestion. These digestive enzymes are produced in the liver from cholesterol. Hence, any binding of these acids leads to a beneficial removal from the body via the stool.

A 1995 study in the *Annals of Internal Medicine*[25] found that 2.5 grams of colestipol plus 2.5 grams of psyllium three times daily before meals was better tolerated and as effective as 5 grams of colestipol alone. The ratio of total cholesterol to high-density lipoprotein (HDL) cholesterol was reduced by 18% with the combination therapy; by little more than 10% with colestipol alone, and by 6 % with psyllium alone (5 grams three times a day). A placebo effect was not active, as the placebo reduced the cholesterol ratio by only 0.1%.

Similarly, studies have shown that

psyllium also enhances the effect of the cholesterol-lowering medication, cholestyramine. One 1997 study in the *Journal of Lipid Research*[26] showed that total bile acid elimination increased by 26% with psyllium alone, 57% with cholestyramine alone, and a whopping 79% by the combination of the two.

Suggested mechanisms for psyllium's cholesterol-lowering effects include 1) its binding of bile acids and 2) the fiber's formation (with water) into a mucilaginous gel that combines with and hinders absorption of the intestinal contents in general (including cholesterol-containing foods). This psyllium-food mixture diminishes the exposed surface area available strictly for food absorption, whether the contents be beneficial (food nutrients, medications) or deleterious (cholesterol). See **Figures 2.1 and 2.2**.

In addition, many fibers (more insoluble than soluble) enhance transit time through the intestine, also impairing absorption of various substances, both good and bad.

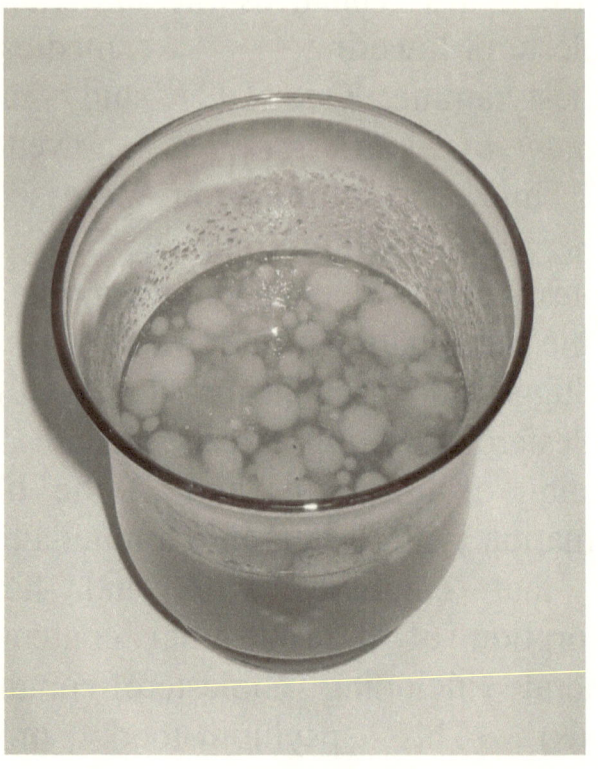

Figure 2.1 Butter floating on top of psyllium-water mixture—before stirring

By the same processes already noted, ingestion of various fibers reduce the digestion and absorption of glucose and various starches, benefiting diabetics. Many soluble fibers also aid diabetics by spreading out the time over which glucose is absorbed, helping to reduce both the incidence of hyper- and hypoglycemia.[27] [28] Any weight loss incurred by fiber's enhanced feeling of satiety and fullness in overweight patients is an added plus.[29]

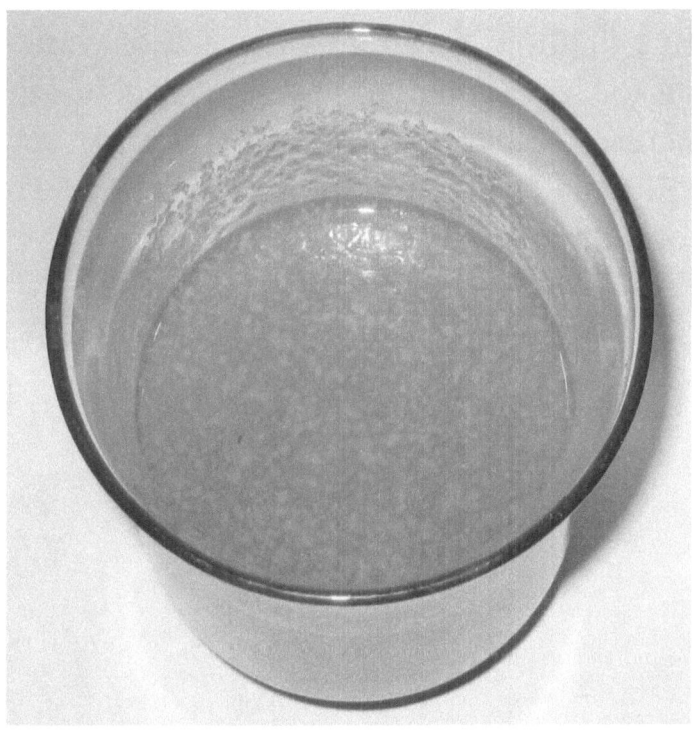

Figure 2.2 Butter after being stirred into psyllium-water mixture

Concerns that some people may voice regarding the risk of diarrhea from various forms of dietary fiber are overblown. The rate of introduction of fiber into the diet is the key to avoiding diarrhea—acclimatize the bowel *gradually*. I for one can attest that the virgin bowel *will* become acclimatized to the fiber. The period of time required for this indoctrination varies, but once the naïve bowel adapts to the increased fiber load, intestinal transit times will usually moderate to a normal or near-normal pace.

Chapter 3: Ready to Add Fiber?

K eep in mind, that despite any negative connotations, the addition of fiber to the diet reestablishes the more "normal" environment from which our bodies have evolved. For those concerned about the absorption of beneficial nutrients and vitamins, this fear can be addressed in a variety of ways. First, any healthy individual on no medications and consuming a well-balanced diet has little to fear. The normal absorption of essential vitamins and minerals in a healthy diet should not be sufficiently reduced to cause any noteworthy deficiencies. Having said that, you should still consult your family doctor and any specialist physicians before adding fiber to your diet. Second, as is commonly recommended for concerned individuals or their physicians, you may simply supplement your diet with a daily multivitamin.

It is also advisable that psyllium and other soluble fibers be taken with plenty of fluids, especially if just sprinkled on or mixed directly with solid foods. The latter is my preferred mode of ingestion for the non-flavored psyllium products. I like to sprinkle and mix the powder in salads, oatmeal, mashed potatoes, pasta, rice, etc. If anyone adopts this practice, make sure you drink plenty of non-alcoholic liquid, preferably a minimum of two 8 ounce glasses per 3.4 g of psyllium husk and a minimum total of 6 glasses per day. Drinking plenty of water with the psyllium will allow the resulting gelatinous mixture to remain liquid enough so that it can travel easily and comfortably through the intestine. A lack of sufficient fluids has the adverse potential of forming an unpleasant, constipating mass within the intestinal tract. In some rare settings, this may even form an obstruction. It is through psyllium's ability to absorb additional fluids that makes it a safe alternative for treating some forms of diarrhea.

Because of these potential risks, however, psyllium manufacturers are now required to have a warning on their labels similar to the following:

Taking this product without adequate fluid may cause it to swell and block your throat or esophagus and may cause choking. Do not take this product if you have difficulty in swallowing. If you experience chest pain, vomiting, or difficulty in swallowing or breathing after taking this product, seek immediate medical attention.[30]

A wheat product known as Benefiber is a wheat dextrin and is actively competing against psyllium in the marketplace. Benefiber is made up of a natural soluble fiber that is advertised as flavorless, dissolves completely in water, and "won't thicken." The product has approximately half the fiber (1.5 gm) per teaspoon as psyllium (3.4 gm per tsp.). Hence, you have to take twice the amount (2 teaspoons) for a full 3-gram fiber dose. Although I could not find any medical studies performed on this or other wheat dextrin products, it is not clear whether the future will reveal that this form of soluble fiber has the same lipid-lowering benefits as psyllium and oat fiber. Its lack of "thickening" or gel formation may well nullify the beneficial affects. This has yet to be determined.

Oatmeal (oat fiber) is another excellent source of soluble fiber and contains about four grams of fiber (half as soluble and half as insoluble fiber) per half cup of the *dry* oats (40 grams).

Probably the most common form of oatmeal is rolled ("old fashioned") oats. Oats, like most cereal grains, have a hard outer husk (chaff) that is usually removed before the grain is eaten. Rolled oats are oats that have subsequently been rolled into flat flakes by heavy rollers. Most forms of commercial oatmeal have been lightly baked or pressure-cooked. "Quick" or "instant" oatmeals are rolled oats that have been chopped up to allow them to absorb water easier and cook faster. Rolled oats are the main ingredient used to make granola. They are an excellent source of thiamine and iron, as well as fiber. Like psyllium, oat fiber is also useful in reducing cholesterol. Oats are additionally an excellent source of antioxidants (that help protect against atherosclerosis) and beta-glucans (useful in type 2 diabetics).

I have found what I consider to be a unique (what many consider unorthodox) and most tasteful way to enjoy rolled oats. Don't cook the oats! I like to pour a bowl of the "oven toasted, old-fashioned" oats straight out of the container, sprinkle them with cinnamon, and perhaps even add a teaspoon of non-flavored psyllium. I then add 1-2 cups of low-fat milk for a nutty and chewy treat. I commonly make this the main building block of my daily lunch and have yet to grow tired of it. For variety, you may add any number of fruits or yogurt instead of cinnamon—and even nuts. Like other foods, you are limited only by your imagination. For a variety of reasons, I've never been a great fan of the gooey cooked oatmeal commonly mixed with sugar and cream.

Dry oats (mixed in some liquid) offer one other advantage over cooked oats. The uncooked product contains substantially more nutrients per volume. Most of the vitamins and minerals in a cup of dry oats are more than double that which is contained in the cooked product. Granted, much of this difference is explicable from the swelling of the oat grain after boiling in water as well as from the cooking process itself. Hence, you can use this to your advantage. By eating the oats uncooked, for instance in cold milk, they will swell somewhat in the stomach and further increase your fullness and satiation— before you eat that entire burger! As with other soluble fibers, *always* take with sufficient liquid (especially if you add extra fiber to the mix).

I give one potential word of caution should you decide to eat any rolled oatmeal product uncooked as described above. Make sure that the oats you purchase have been "oven-toasted," "roasted," steamed (traditional "rolled oats"), or otherwise processed to kill any bacteria. Although most processors routinely do this (typical for the rolled oats sold on most store shelves), this is not the norm for all types of oatmeal, including *steel-cut* oats for instance. For steel-cut oats, this is probably not a great concern since these oats require boiling for a minimum of about 20-30 minutes just to be able to eat (chew) them. To be safe, however, check out that your brand of particular oats have been sterilized in some manner. The Internet or any 800 #s on the product label should serve to answer any questions.

My recommendation for initiating these fibers into your diet are now described.

As previously noted, I recommend the Institute of Medicine's simple dosage suggestion of at least 14 grams of fiber for every 1000 calories consumed.[31]

You can also plan your intake and ratio of soluble to insoluble fiber based upon any specific needs you are addressing. For most extra-colonic issues (e.g., diabetes, cardiovascular, and cancer risks) and the *inflammatory* bowel ailments, most authorities suggest taking predominantly soluble fiber. For the prevention of diverticular disease and constipation, they recommend mainly insoluble fiber. To address multiple concerns, you may need to take a combination of the two. Consult with your physician.

I wish to re-emphasize that your fiber intake should be increased *gradually*. Slow down if your bowel habits change too drastically. For problems with constipation (rare), increase your fluid intake and/or insoluble fibers. For problems with diarrhea, decrease your insoluble fibers and/or increase your soluble fibers. You may then continue with the addition of extra fiber once your bowels have adjusted to the increased load. This may take weeks or even months. Your digestive system will warn you if you are proceeding too rapidly.

Although I do enjoy the taste of my non-cooked rolled oats, I preferred the ease and convenience (especially with travel) of psyllium. It has several major advantages over the other fibers:

It provides variety and versatility when you are just not in the mood for a cereal bran or you are on the road. (I carry a small container of psyllium religiously in my pocket when I eat out.) You may mix the non-flavored psyllium with the contents of your meal or dissolve it in any *noncarbonated* beverage (carbonated beverages will cause the fiber to fizz out all over the table). I will also use the psyllium when I am in the workplace or out at a public restaurant. When the meal arrives, I sprinkle the powder onto the selected portion of my meal or into my water. I tell curious onlookers that it is my cholesterol "medication."

I need to add one additional point. Do not confuse or compare fiber use with that of any type of general or stimulant laxative. Fiber laxatives fall into a totally different category of product and should never be confused with stimulant laxatives. From a general standpoint, there is very little need for a healthy individual to use any stimulant laxative. In fact, the reverse is true. Stimulant laxatives, especially those of the senna category, can be deleterious to your health to the extent of causing a condition known as colonic inertia ("sluggish bowel") and another malady known as melanosis coli (or "black colon").

On June 4, 2009, as I was researching the various topics for this book, *USA Today* published the aptly titled article "Kellogg adds fiber, hoping to bowl cereal consumers over."[32] Kellogg's, the maker of All-Bran, had just announced that by the end of 2010, eighty percent of its cereals would contain at least 3 grams of fiber per serving. Neither the article nor the Internet named the type of fiber to be used. Still, this was a giant leap for the health of humankind, particularly children since the Kellogg's cereals to be targeted were those for kids. The article went on to imply that the addition of fiber to various foods had become quite fashionable, and it named other companies which had already added fiber to their products. They included Dannon (Activa), Kraft (Wheat Thins Fiber Selects, and, due out in January 2010, Fiber Fit granola bars and cookies), and Frito-Lay (SmartFood Popcorn Clusters).

Keep in mind that, although these fiber additions represent an improvement, some of these products still contain some significant unwanted ingredients. Hence, continue to read the nutrition facts of all products and choose accordingly.

For those consuming fiber for any

reason, the fiber should always be taken with meals to allow the fiber to mix with the food to enhance its overall health benefits. Be sure to take your dietary fiber, supplemental vitamins, and any necessary medications around the time schedules recommended by your physician.

Chapter 4: A Summary of Fiber's Many Benefits

Of all the Western world's modern maladies, constipation must rank as one of the most prevalent, due almost entirely from the low dietary fiber consumption of the developed nations.

Although our harried life styles and social demands constrain us to limit our bathroom time to a minimum, our low dietary fiber consumption only serves to promote this unhealthy practice—at our bowel's expense. Hard stools lead to straining. Straining leads to hemorrhoids, anal fissures (tears), and diverticular disease. Before you know it, you're hooked on laxatives or under the knife for a hemorrhoidectomy, bleeding diverticulum, perforated colon, or worse.

Although dietary fiber may not come

with any guarantees, I am convinced that any unpleasant side effects, though few (e.g., gas, loose stools), are worth any short-term inconvenience. The long-term benefits are worth the effort: An incomplete list follows:

1. Insoluble, "bulk" fibers are successfully used to treat/prevent constipation, hemorrhoids, anal fissures (caused by large hard stools), diverticulosis and the complications of diverticular disease, and obesity.

2. Soluble fibers are used to treat a number of conditions, including certain diarrheal conditions (e.g., by absorbing water), irritable bowel syndrome (involving both diarrhea and constipation), hemorrhoids, anal fissures (caused by the chronic irritation of frequent diarrhea), inflammatory bowel diseases, high cholesterol, heart disease, diabetes, and obesity.

3. Further studies appear necessary to better define the exact role of fiber in the prevention of cancers of the

gastrointestinal tract, prostate, breast, and uterus.

There exists substantial overlap between the many benefits of both soluble and insoluble fibers. Oats, for example, are almost exactly half soluble and half insoluble fiber. Nature has undoubtedly selected such ratios for a reason. For the average individual, each fiber type offers a valued assortment of select advantages, and a combination of the two is recommended. For other conditions, however, one fiber type may be more appropriate.

As always, seek your physician's advice before adding any type of fiber to your diet—including when you take the fiber in relationship to meals and your medications.

Chapter 5: Alternative Therapies and Health Measures

In the field of medicine, physicians have seen it all, and it is unusual to shock a seasoned practitioner. Having said that, it saddens many of us as medical doctors to see products that claim to perform a number of ridiculous feats within the human body. The "cleansing" of various organs is just one such example. I have yet to read of any reputable medical studies to substantiatc any of these claims.

The closest thing to a "cleansing" of any bodily organ is the topic of this book, whereby the ingestion of *natural* dietary fibers conveys a bevy of healthful properties to the bowel and, in turn, its proprietor. I also interject that this practice (ingesting dietary fiber) is not truly a cleansing at all. Instead, fiber merely maintains the ideal intestinal milieu for proper functioning of this all-important organ system. The ingestion of dietary fibers represents a simple means of achieving and maintaining your bowel (and bodily) health.

It is only because we humans have slipped into such deplorable health practices (or absence thereof) that we even need to consider the option of "cleansing" any of our organ systems. It is a sad state of affairs. In the words of an excerpt from WebMD:

What you eat—not what you flush through your colon—may have the greatest impact on colon health, lowering your risk of colon cancer and enhancing your overall health.

Increasing both soluble and insoluble fiber can help with a wide range of gastrointestinal problems, including constipation, diverticular disease, and colorectal cancer....

Be aware, if the therapist adds a substance to the water during colon irrigation, you run the risk of an allergic reaction. Do not use laxatives or colon irrigations long term. They can irritate or upset the balance of your colon's good bacteria and interfere with normal bowel function. [33]

Most physicians recommend that you avoid colon irrigations, if you have any of the following conditions:

1. Diverticulitis
2. Ulcerative colitis
3. Crohn's disease
4. Severe hemorrhoids
5. Tumors in your rectum or colon
6. Recent bowel surgery
7. Heart disease or kidney disease, unless approved by your health care provider. [34]

WebMD then goes on to list the potential side effects and complications of colon irrigations:

1. Vomiting, nausea, cramps
2. Dizziness, a sign of dehydration
3. Mineral imbalance

4. Potential interference with medication absorption on day of procedure
5. Bowel perforation
6. Infection
7. Depletion of helpful normal bowel flora unless replaced (i.e. probiotics)[35]

The same site notes that our bodies are already capable, without "detoxifying" or "cleansing" irrigations, of the following natural processes:

1. Natural bacteria in the colon detoxify food wastes.
2. The liver neutralizes toxins.
3. Mucus membranes in the colon keep unwanted substances from reentering the blood and tissues.
4. The colon sheds old cells about every 3 days, preventing a buildup of harmful material...[36]

Yet, it is the reality of life in our modern age that we wish to mitigate our unhealthy lifestyles by doing something. However, in the wise words of Hippocrates, "First, do no harm." In this light, let us examine the benefits, as well as the consequences, of several alternative practices and products.

Enemas

The introduction of liquids into the rectum and colon has existed since the 17th century when large syringes (without the needle) were used to introduce fluid into the rectum.

The introduction of liquid into the rectum and colon expands the bowel lumen and causes a potent reflexive contraction. With the liquid's additional lubricant effects, a resultant and effective evacuation of the entire lower colon is not unusual. This constipation remedy has definite advantages over oral laxatives or rectal suppositories in its effectiveness and speed.

Throughout history, the types of liquids utilized for flooding the rectum for this purpose have spanned a wide gamut and been limited only by the creativity of the administrator—not always to the patient's benefit. The fluids have included but not been limited to isotonic saline (the least irritating) to the rectum and colon, plain water, water with baking soda (sodium bicarbonate), water with a mild soap, buffered sodium phosphate, mineral oil, glycerol, and even "home" mixtures utilizing molasses and milk.

From the information we have already reviewed, it is not hard to imagine some of the unintended consequences of these remedies. Potential side effects include the following, sometimes with lethal consequences:

1. Plain water may either draw electrolytes from the bloodstream (into the colon) or the reverse: dilution of the blood through its absorption of the water. The consequences are similar: constituents (e.g., electrolytes) in the blood will decrease.
2. Water with baking soda may absorb water from the bloodstream, raising the level of blood constituents (e.g., electrolytes).

3. Buffered sodium phosphate solutions may also draw water from the bloodstream and will stimulate colonic contractions.
4. Mineral oil, although relatively safe and effective, may continue to leak from the patient's hindside for up to 24 hours.
5. Certain soaps mixed in water can irritate the rectum and cause a chemical colitis.
6. Inappropriately administered enemas may result in bowel perforation and/or infection.

Some people utilize enemas, not just for the intended relief of constipation and fecal impaction, but also for a host of cleansing applications: e.g., for accepted cleansings prior to some medical exams (such as colonoscopies) or, conversely, for alternative medicine "detoxifications" (already discussed). As noted, there is scanty to zero evidence that colonic irrigations in the healthy person serve any beneficial purpose. As with anything else in medicine, unnecessary, though seemingly benign procedures may, on occasion, invite risks as noted above.

In recent history, the enema has also served medically as a vehicle for the administration of fluids for rehydration (when intravenous therapy is unavailable or not applicable), certain medications, and even "recreational" drugs of abuse.

As with any other medical practice, your family physician can advise you as to the wisdom and appropriateness of the enema in your particular situation.

Fecal transplants

If you have never heard the term "fecal transplant," the wording probably causes a variety of unpleasant mental images to arise. Unfortunately, as unpleasant as these images might be, they are probably accurate.

Also referred to as fecal bacteriotherapy, fecal transfusion, stool transplant, fecal enema, and human probiotic infusion, the first known fecal transplant was performed by merely having the recipient drink a milkshake impregnated with someone else's pureed feces. This technique is not far removed from the mechanism replicated by nature. The newborn typically receives her first "injection" of gut microorganisms through the oral introduction (yes, by mouth) of the mother's fecal bacteria (more crudely, her feces) released during the normal process of vaginal delivery.

During vaginal delivery, the mother invariably expels feces during the pushing maneuver that also propels the fetus through the vaginal canal. As you will see, as disgusting as this may sound, nature knows what's best.

The most challenging question for physicians has now evolved, not in how the newborn receives her first gut flora (it's by mouth) but how the baby delivered by the sterile technique of C-section does.

At birth, the microbial content of the newborn is essentially sterile until it becomes colonized via the environment. The options are essentially two-fold for the newborn baby. It can receive the preponderance of its bowel bacteria from the mother (e.g., through vaginal delivery and breast feeding) and/or indirectly via the surrounding environment (i.e., all those things the newborn stuffs into its mouth—sanctioned and otherwise). One can only imagine the possibilities.

The fact that so many C-section babies survive their infancies with few, if any, ill effects attests to the prevalence of normal human intestinal bacteria all around us and within our vast and varied surroundings.

The fact that the human body has so successfully evolved, immersed within this bacterial-laden milieu, attests to the recently documented disadvantages of many modern attempts to sterilize our surrounding. Cleanliness, it appears, is only good up to a point. Certainly the demarcation is unclear, but multiple studies suggest that a total abstinence of "dirt" exposure for the baby's developing immune system has the potential for future problems as adults, with allergies being the predominant manifestation detected to date.

Medical studies have documented that babies delivered by C-section (as well as babies fed mainly formula instead of breast milk, by the way) have substantially different and fewer of the beneficial bacteria within their intestines than babies delivered vaginally (and breast fed).

It is conceivable that pediatricians may soon start recommending that future infants delivered by C-section start receiving fecal transplants from their mothers.

Currently, due to society's reticence to accept such a disturbing medical technique, especially via the oral route (though simple, inexpensive, and medically acceptable—with caveats), the medical community suggests that fecal transplants be accomplished via the more agreeable rectal route: enema—with the "sample" obtained from a healthy human donor. "Healthy" and "human" are the key words here.

As with so many procedures in medicine, the rectal regimen greatly increases the complexity, cost, and length of administration. Some bolder doctors (with a more liberal patient population perhaps) may employ the simpler and more cost-effective nasogastric-tube route—still more expensive than the milk-shake technique.

Because of (not-surprising) public reluctance, most physicians restrict the fecal transplant procedure (sadly) to patients suffering only from potentially fatal illnesses. At the time of this writing, the procedure is advocated primarily for patients with refractory *Clostridium difficile* infection (a severe form of diarrhea), but the procedure has also proven effective for select types of colitis, constipation, irritable bowel syndrome, and even some neurological disorders (e.g., multiple sclerosis, Parkinson's disease, and myoclonus dystonia[37]). The mechanisms for the improvement seen in many of these diseases is poorly understood. We may conclude, however, that our gut flora appears to harbor more importance to our overall health than we have ever believed.

In addition, fecal transplantation appears to be extraordinarily effective. In *Clostridium difficile* infection, for instance, where restoring the normal flora of the bowel is all that is required, patients often recover after only a single treatment.

We continue to learn and be amazed.

The Valsalva maneuver

Named after a 17th century physician (Antonio Maria Valsalva) in Italy, the Valsalva maneuver is the act of attempting to expel air ("pushing") against a closed airway. This forceful action is frequently employed to evacuate the rectum (or vagina during childbirth) of its contents.

This commonly employed maneuver, however, places undue strain on the cardiovascular system as well as its intended rectal target. Blood pressure will typically increase in proportion to the amount of strain applied.

A normal bodily reflex from any sudden rise in blood vessel pressure often triggers the heart to dramatically decrease its rate of contractions (the heart rate). This reflex is known as the *vasovagal reflex*. If the heart rate slows enough, the person may pass out: vasovagal syncope. Certain individuals are more susceptible to this bodily response and will testify to the sensation of lightheadedness (or history of syncope) brought about by this activity.

More lethal consequences to the Valsalva are stroke or even death, caused from the effects of a disastrous rise in blood pressure. As with any type of stroke, high blood pressure will endanger the rupture of a brain aneurysm or risk dislodging a blood clot.

Knowledge and caution are the modalities for avoiding such consequences of simply wishing to evacuate your bowels. Certainly fiber helps to ease the act of expelling one's feces, but I have already emphasized the importance of this point.

My personal recommendation is to modify the Valsalva by never completely closing your airway (glottis). You can "push" against a partially closed airway (and slowly exhaling) to greatly reduce these potential risks. In addition, utilizing more of your abdominal muscles to help evacuate the rectum, as opposed to the Valsalva alone, is a free form of exercise, accessible without travel to a fitness center.

Rare but conceivable adverse side effects of fiber

1. Any health supplements, including fiber, should only be taken under a physician's supervision. *Some patients should not take specific fibers.*
2. Fiber supplements may diminish, delay, or otherwise alter absorption of certain medications, thereby altering their actions. Some of the most problematic interactions include lithium containing drugs, certain types of antidepressants, and various diabetic, seizure, and heart medications. Always seek your physician's recommendations. Most physicians will advise taking approved oral medications at least 1 (one) hour *before* or at least 2 (two) hours *after* the fiber.
3. Always follow the manufacturers' guidelines for taking fiber

supplements. For example, mixing psyllium improperly in insufficient fluid can make it difficult (and problematic for some) to swallow. With the ingestion of any fiber supplement, always be sure to accompany the fiber with adequate (physician-approved)   fluids: typically 8 ounces at the time of taking each supplement, with a daily *total* fluid intake of at least 6 (8-ounce) glasses.

4. If you develop any bodily pain (especially chest or abdominal), difficulty swallowing, or shortness of breath after taking fiber, seek immediate medical attention—good advice even if you're not taking fiber. As with any health supplement, allergic reactions always exist as potential complications.

Anal Hygiene

Proper care of the oft-neglected anus includes recommendations that most humans find despicable and prefer to avoid…usually at all costs. I recommend actually touching and washing—*in and around* the anus—and preferably as soon as possible after each bowel movement. I realize that this ideal is not practical when you're at the workplace or other public areas.

Let's face it, the anus takes more than its fair share of abuse. The most unsanitary act of the entire human body occurs within its purview…and we return the favor with only a couple of swipes of folded tissue followed by neglect—at least until the next time nature calls.

Even in the event of an unusually hardened passage of fecal material or an otherwise resistant bowel movement, we refuse to alter our regimen. Small tears or cracks (fissures) within the anal ring fester inside this extremely contaminated milieu. It is surprising that infections in and around the anus (including any highly vascular hemorrhoids) don't occur more frequently. Really, the anus deserves better.

If physicians can probe patients' rectums on a daily basis and survive, then so can we. As noxious as cleaning the anus might appear, the payoff is well worth it. I recommend lathering your hands well with a mild hand soap and gently (preferably with short nails) cleanse the entire anal area and introduce a well-lathered finger into the anal ring (and yes, with likely penetration into the rectal lumen). The soap will serve a dual purpose as a valuable lubricant as well as a cleanser. Your finger does not have to remain within the confines of the ring for long—just long enough to clean (and then subsequently to rinse) the anal canal. While your finger is doing its job, you may wish to take note of the normal anatomy of this area for future reference—to allow you to detect future changes should any develop. There is no real need to do a full pelvic or prostate exam.

When first instituting this practice, you will need to overcome the initial shock of seeing fecal material on your hands. Get over it. Your body is literally seething with bacteria. If you're seeking to avoid bacterial contamination, it's too late. Your body and its most intimate surfaces are already seething with bacteria.

The final part to the cleaning process, not to be overlooked, is to repeat the former steps with warm tap water so as to rinse the areas you have just cleaned, including the entire anal ring area. For obvious reasons, a shower offers the best venue for cleaning and rinsing the anus— as opposed to a bath. As noted in one Seinfeld episode, you don't want to be "sitting there in a tepid pool of [your] own filth."

For women, rinsing is of special importance, and females want to avoid direct contamination of the female genitalia. The short length of the female urethra already predisposes itself to urinary tract infections (UTI's). This latter risk goes both ways—neglected anal hygiene places females at just as high a risk as improper washings. Physicians recommend that women should always wipe and clean utilizing front-to-back motions.

The benefits of proper anal hygiene can not be overstated. Not only might you significantly reduce your incidence of anal abscesses and infected and thrombosed hemorrhoids, but consistent palpation and knowledge of your own personal anatomy, much like doing your own breast and testicular exams, will allow you to detect early, serious abnormalities like anal cancer (which can occur in even young patients, including one case that I diagnosed early in my own medical practice).

Remember, "cleanliness is next to Godliness" (Charles Dickens, Chapter 4: *Great Expectations*).

Chapter 6: Hyperacidity

The prevalence of stomach problems in the general population is probably greater than 15%, if not higher. Dyspepsia is a generic term for indigestion and describes any host of maladies identified by gastroesophageal reflux disease (or GERD, stomach acid spilling into the esophagus), gastritis (stomach inflammation), or even peptic ulcer disease (mucosal erosions in the stomach, duodenum, or esophagus).

Any or all of these conditions and their respective treatments may affect the sanctity of the remaining intestine and is why I have opted to include this chapter in the text of a book focused on the colon.

It would appear that you are either predisposed to stomach conditions involving hyperacidity or you're not. I have had the condition all my life. In contrast, I have never known my wife to have an episode of heartburn.

Although the above stomach-related afflictions typically cause their *symptoms* through the highly irritating and erosive effects of stomach acid, the actual *cause* of each disorder can vary widely and include the likes of anatomic abnormalities (e.g., a poorly functioning lower esophageal sphincter), pathologic bacteria (*Helicobacter pylori*), medications (aspirin and the nonsteroidal anti-inflammatory drugs), alcohol, or even cancer. As such, it is up to you and your physician to devise appropriate treatment plans for your specific condition.

Yet, despite our best laid plans, we often find ourselves having to deal with the severity of these conditions in a variety of awkward social settings, while travelling, or at 3:00 a.m. in the morning. Hence, it is always convenient to have a handful of options available.

For healthy patients without any cardiovascular disease (including high blood pressure), simple bicarbonate of soda (sodium bicarbonate, baking soda) is greatly underutilized. Due to its high sodium content, it should never be used in patients with high blood pressure, congestive heart failure, renal disease, or other edematous states. Due to its inherent property of being an *absorbable* antacid, it may predispose some patients to electrolyte abnormalities and alkalosis. Even healthy patients should avoid taking sodium bicarbonate above the recommended dosage.

Another problem may arise if sodium bicarb is taken with calcium containing products and foods (e.g., dairy) because of a complication known as the *milk-alkali syndrome* which may provoke kidney stones, kidney failure, and tissue calcium deposition. This syndrome got its name, like it sounds, from patients who repeatedly ingested absorbable antacids with milk.

On an empty stomach, sodium bicarb is safe for most healthy patients when taken as directed. Manufacturer Arm and Hammer recommends taking ½ teaspoon of their product, mixed in ½ glass of water, as needed "every 2 hours, or as directed by a physician" for heartburn and acid indigestion. What I particularly like about this product is that it is inexpensive, highly effective, and works almost immediately. If you don't get relief within 10-15 minutes, you should try something else or call a doctor. The main immediate side effect is temporary belching from the carbon dioxide produced ($NaHCO_3$ + HCl $\rightarrow$ $\underline{\mathbf{CO_2}}$ + H2O + NaCl).

Oddly, as safe as sodium bicarbonate is for healthy individuals, the same cannot be said for the even more popular antacid products containing calcium, especially calcium carbonate (e.g., Tums and Rolaids). These popular antacids *do* immediately relieve heartburn…but calcium stimulates stomach acid production. Thus, many people, although experiencing immediate heartburn relief, will undergo a calcium-related rebound in hyperacidity later,[38] and a vicious cycle sets in. For this reason as a physician, I seldom recommend calcium-containing antacids for heartburn.

Several of my favorite antacids, however, are Pepto-Bismol (Procter and

Gamble) and two *liquid* products, Maalox (Novartis International AG) and Mylanta (by McNeil Consumer Healthcare, a subsidiary of Johnson and Johnson). [Note, this section discusses only the liquid versions of Maalox and Mylanta. I do not recommend the tablets because they contain quite different ingredients from the liquids.]

Pepto-Bismol and its generic counterparts act by quite different mechanisms than Maalox/Mylanta and their generics.[39] [By the way, I have found the generic products to be just as effective as the name brands and, of course, are far less expensive.]

Pepto-Bismol's active ingredient is bismuth subsalicylate. Researchers believe that this bismuth compound acts through several mechanisms. The product stimulates the stomach to produce protective mucus and bicarbonate. The bismuth also inhibits a digestive enzyme (pepsin), and a bismuth byproduct collects in the base of erosive ulcers, speeding their healing. Lastly, bismuth possesses an antibacterial action against *H. pylori*. For an over-the-counter (OTC) product with no direct antacid activity, this product is very safe and effective.

Researchers estimate that only about 1% of oral bismuth is actually absorbed because the poorly water-soluble product is converted to insoluble bismuth byproducts in the stomach. On the other hand, the salicylate portion of the bismuth molecule is absorbed to the tune of greater than 90%. As such, and since the typical adult dose of the standard (not maximum or double strength) product is two tablespoons and contains 262 mg of bismuth subsalicylate per tbsp., you will be ingesting the equivalent of 524 mg of salicylate. The standard aspirin tablet contains 325 mg of acetyl-salicylate, so you will, in essence, be taking just less than the standard equivalent dose of aspirin per standard dose of Pepto-Bismol. For this reason, patients who cannot take aspirin (bleeding risks, on anticoagulants, allergy to aspirin, or may have Reye's syndrome) should not take Pepto-Bismol.

Patients should also note that bismuth turns the stools (and sometimes tongue) black (harmless), which may be confused with blood in the stool. Hence, Pepto-Bismol is best taken when you and your doctor believe you are not at a risk for any gastrointestinal bleeding.

Pepto-Bismol is also somewhat constipating and may, therefore, serve as a treatment for diarrhea. Because of this constipating effect, I take only half the recommended dose (e.g., one tablespoon), and supplement the missing portion with a balancing half-dose (two teaspoons) of either of the liquids Maalox or Mylanta, which are mild laxatives because of the magnesium hydroxide (Milk of Magnesia) they contain.

Both liquids of the standard (not maximum or double) strength Maalox and Mylanta contain 200mg aluminum hydroxide, 200mg magnesium hydroxide, and 20 mg of a nonabsorbable antigas agent, simethicone,[40] per teaspoon.

Both aluminum hydroxide and magnesium hydroxide are efficient and relatively nonabsorbable antacids. Magnesium hydroxide has the side effects of being a mild laxative and may disturb iron and folic acid absorption. Aluminum hydroxide, on the other hand, like bismuth, is mildly constipating. Hence, the magnesium and aluminum hydroxides counterbalance each other relatively well as far as their effects on the bowel go. I have noticed—personal experience—that the laxative effect of the magnesium seems to slightly outweigh the constipating effects of the aluminum hydroxide. For this reason, the addition of a bismuth subsalicylate product adds further benefit to both the stomach and bowel.

As with any drug, and no matter how benign these various products are for healthy individuals, they can still cause potential problems in certain disease states—or from overuse. The potential risks include kidney damage, high serum magnesium (especially in-patients with kidney disease), and low blood phosphate (the aluminum hydroxide will bind with serum phosphates).

As with any other medication (OTC or prescription), there is always the potential of an allergic reaction (rash, swelling, difficulty breathing), for which immediate medical treatment needs to be sought. As with so many medications, they may interfere with the actions or absorption of other drugs (e.g., digoxin, iron, and certain antibiotics, including the tetracyclines and ciprofloxacin, to name a few).

Yet, despite the fore-mentioned precautions, these drugs have a proven safety record in healthy individuals.

For people who, for whatever medical reasons, cannot take the above OTC medications, the medical field offers a host of other options—any of which are better than a perforated, bleeding ulcer. Again, your physician will be able to recommend the options which are best for you.

When I personally need to resort to more potent drugs for my own problematic stomach, I prefer the use of a class of proven drugs known as the proton pump inhibitors (PPIs). This group of relatively recent acid inhibitors (both OTC and prescription) is currently one of the most popular and widely sold group of drugs in the world. These drugs are beneficial for a whole host of ailments whose problems center around stomach acid production, including the likes of GERD, peptic ulcer disease, or just simple dyspepsia.

The PPIs act by blocking the proton (acidic hydrogen ion) generators ("pumps") of the gastric acid-producing parietal cells and must be absorbed into the bloodstream to be effective.

This class of drugs is significantly more effective than the older H2-class of acid antagonist drugs. The PPIs may reduce stomach acid secretion by up to 99%.

The PPI-induced reduction of stomach acid aids in the rapid healing of acid-related erosions and ulcerations. Despite their effectiveness, the improper or prolonged use of these drugs may cause a condition called hypochlorhydria, the lack of sufficient stomach or hydrochloric acid, HCl, production.

Regardless of all the negatives surrounding stomach acid, we could not live without it. Stomach acid is a necessary requirement for the proper digestion of our ingested foods and the vital absorption of many nutrients, particularly vitamin B12 and calcium. Hence, overuse can result in vitamin B12 deficiency, low calcium, bone fractures, heart arrhythmias, and even low serum magnesium.

Allergic reactions are always a potential danger (with any medication), and a special risk from PPI overuse is the development of certain infections. Stomach acid, unbeknownst to many, acts as a wonderfully protective mechanism against ingested bacteria. In the absence or lowering of stomach acid, our bodies are more susceptible to intestinal infections (e.g., *C. difficile* diarrhea) and even some community-acquired pneumonias.

Despite the potential side effects, however, Wikipedia.org notes, "In general, proton pump inhibitors are well tolerated, and the incidence of short-term adverse effects is relatively uncommon."[41]

The long term clinical experience with these drugs has proven their relative safety and value for the many conditions of hyperacidity with which so many of us are afflicted.

Lastly, to end this chapter, I must relate one nearly totally benign treatment that has never failed me—as strange as it may sound: hard candy. No, I'm not kidding.

When I have no access to the above medications—or they have failed me (because I have waited too long to initiate treatment), hard candy always works. My own candy of choice is Skittles, but everyone will have their own favorite.

There is a perfectly valid physiologic explanation for my finding. Human saliva has a pH of between 6.2 and 7.4. The pH of stomach acid, on the other hand, ranges between 1.5 and 3.5. Hard candy, especially tart candies (like Skittles), stimulate significant quantities of saliva. As long as a relatively high pH fluid (saliva) is flowing into a low pH stomach (and also rinsing and neutralizing an irritated lower esophagus for GERD sufferers), relief is typically just a swallow away. Although I cannot guarantee this treatment for everyone, I will repeat that it has never failed me. The downside is obvious: calorie intake. This treatment is not practical for diabetics or persons fighting obesity, unless sugar-free candies are utilized. I have never tried them, but there is no reason that they should not be just as effective. (Beware the risks, if any, of the sugar substitutes used and the quantities you will be ingesting.) Skittles work for me, and I'm not going to mess with success. I do have to adjust my subsequent caloric intake accordingly, however.

Of course, we all know that certain foods and practices are known to cause stomach problems. Some of the greatest offenders are listed below:

1. Alcohol
2. Chocolate
3. Caffeine-containing foods and beverages
4. Calcium
5. High fat and fried foods
6. Some acidic foods like citrus and tomatoes
7. Peppermint
8. Smoking
9. Certain drugs such as the non-steroidal anti-inflammatory drugs (NSAIDs) which include aspirin

The above is far from being a comprehensive list. As always, check with your doctor for any questions and before starting or stopping any medication, even OTCs.

Myths

There is little if any evidence that spices cause stomach irritation. Rather, if your stomach is already inflamed or has erosions from other causes, various spices may impact the raw and exposed nerve endings of the already irritated stomach. In the end though, it is best to avoid any food that consistently causes you heartburn—rational or not.

The discussions in this chapter involving the stomach impact the remainder of the bowel. The stomach just happens to lie more proximal; that's all. The various medications and foods which affect the stomach invariably also affect the remainder of the bowel. A healthy esophagus, stomach, pylorus, and intestine are all part and parcel of a healthy bowel.

Chapter 7: Positions on the Throne

For those who might appreciate any recommendations on how to help to initiate a bowel movement or to enhance a complete evacuation, the following information may prove useful. The human body, according to various scholars, has evolved (think Neanderthal) to do its business in the woods, often in the cold, without the assistance of a modern-day porcelain toilet. As such, our bodies have had to do with what nature has provided—no extras. Evacuation of our bowels, for both male and female, has historically performed best in the squatting position—feet planted firmly with the knees bent and calves touching the back of the thighs. I have witnessed that infants will frequently assume this position for their own evacuations. This is the position, if you believe the evolutionists and medical gastroenterologists, that the human body has perfected over the millennia to help expedite this important bodily function. This positioning of the rectum and sigmoid has theoretically allowed gravity, the increase of intra-abdominal pressure (through hip flexion and the resulting increased pressure applied against the abdomen), and any additional colonic reflexes to work their magic to best eliminate the contents of our bowels.

According to the experts, the introduction of the raised toilet seat has actually distanced us from this preferred evolutionary positioning, and hindered the normal colonic evacuation.

In much of Africa, Asia, and the Middle East, *squatting* toilets are allegedly the norm instead of sitting toilets—although I have never seen one (except pictured in texts), even in my travels to Africa and the Middle East. Individuals supposedly squat on top of the toilet instead of assuming a seated position. The sides are wider to accommodate the feet, and there is no "seat" to raise and lower. Do not attempt this stance on the common (Western) toilet, since there is not an adequate platform upon which to balance the body's weight. Bockus' textbook on *Gastroenterology*[42] actually notes, with this stance, that the thighs press against the abdomen and increase intra-abdominal pressure to aid in the evacuative process.

An Internet search reveals a height for most sitting toilets ranging between 14-16 inches. The toilets in my home ranged from 14.25 to 16.5 inches (not including the hinged seat). For the elderly, this elevation can be raised even more—an extra 6 inches by purchasing an elevated seat to assist in standing up. Needless to say, unless you are a basketball player, most individuals do not come even close to the squatting position when seated on most modern toilets. Shorter individuals are obviously at a greater disadvantage than taller folk in this regard, and they may wish to employ other strategies if difficult bowel evacuations or constipation are an issue.

For a person of average height and weight, a semi-squatting position (without actually having to squat, to be discussed) will in many cases aid an evacuation. Be forewarned: This is not a rapid process and may require faithful patience over many minutes.

The following are simple basic adjustments which you can make to more closely achieve a relative squatting-like position—without actually climbing up onto the stool (not recommended):

1. Elevating the heels of both feet (in a tiptoe-like position) by a couple of inches can assist some with a difficult evacuation. I have noted some moderate success with this simple maneuver. This technique is especially useful when you're away from home and unable to employ #2 below.

2. At home, you can avoid the prolonged positioning of #1 above by merely placing a small platform (e.g., a 4-inch by 4-inch by 2-foot length of lumber) under your feet to elevate your thighs toward the abdomen. Never stand up,

however, while your feet are still on the wooden platform. The platform is meant only to raise your thighs closer to your abdomen. It is not intended nor stable enough to bear your weight.

3. Probably the position of choice: Simply bending forward (with your thighs pressing slightly against the lower abdomen) will help in a large percentage of cases (**Figure 7.1**).

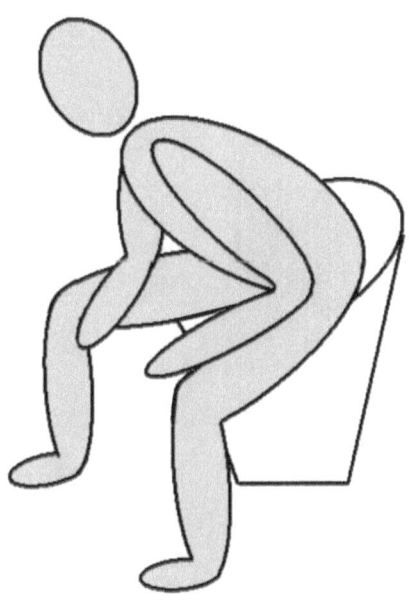

Figure 7.1 Bending forward

For thin individuals, placement of the forearms between the upper thighs and lower abdomen (with hands folded between your knees, for example) should provide adequate added pressure to the abdomen (**Figure 7.2**).

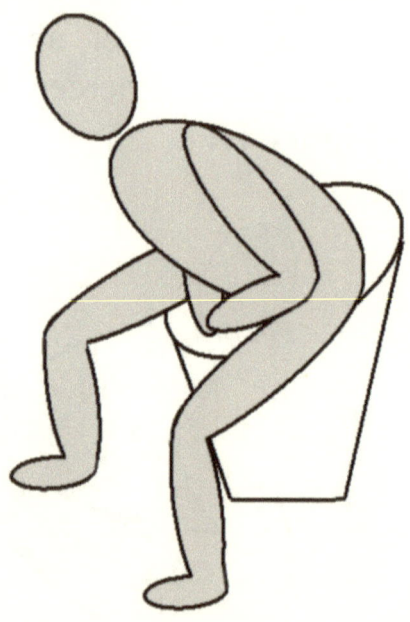

Figure 7.2 Forearms between thighs and abdomen

I have found this simple bending-forward maneuver to be the easiest and the most effective in aiding many difficult evacuations, though the positioning may take notable time to prompt the necessary colonic reflexes and related mechanics into action. A good book or magazine is always helpful since you can't expect to rush Mother Nature. Additionally, do not become discouraged if you note passage of flatus instead of a bowel movement. Rather than being a false alarm, the flatus may instead signal the movement of gas ahead of a fecal bolus from higher up in the bowel, simply making its slow way down into the sigmoid and, eventually, the rectum. If there has been no activity after 30 minutes, however, you should consider that the sensation of fullness may be a false alarm (e.g., flatus) or that added measures (e.g., an enema) might prove helpful.

4. Should the above simple measures fail you, and you wish to implement a squatting toilet without having to actually buy and install one, some

enterprising dealers sell adaptive supports that surround the front of the modern toilet to allow you to squat over the bowl rather than sit—transforming the bowl into a veritable squatting toilet. This last option is a less expensive choice for those not interested in purchasing and installing a true squatter.

Note: Any case of either acute and severe or chronic constipation requires a physician's attention and evaluation to rule out treatable causes.

As noted in the preceding chapters, avoid the Valsalva maneuver during bowel movements, including difficult evacuations. If you believe additional straining is necessary, I recommend only a minimal but constant tightening of the abdominal muscles, without straining against a closed windpipe. Tightening of the abdomen, even slightly but for a constant interval, may greatly assist movement of a fecal bolus (if such material is present in the lower colon) toward the area of lower pressure in the rectum. This practice also proves beneficial, as does any healthful isometric exercise.

Certainly our bowel evacuations are highly personalized and individualized. Every individual, just as with anything in life and medicine, is very different—plus each situation regarding one's bowels varies on a daily basis. A position which proved useful yesterday is not necessarily going to be helpful today. Leaning backward may be as beneficial today as leaning forward proved useful yesterday.

The human body is predictably unpredictable. I read one amusing Internet account where a man professed to aid his daily evacuations by raising his hands up over his head! Hence, the advice offered in this section may or may not prove useful to everyone.

Chapter 8: Conclusions

In ending, I want to respond to several questions that I have received over the years regarding fiber and types of bran. Following are some of the more frequent questions I have been asked:

1. Q: I want to eat a fiber that won't give me gas.
   A: Unfortunately, nearly any soluble fiber will generate gas as the bacteria in the lower intestines ferment its various constituents (mainly the oligosaccharides). This is why beans have garnished their ill repute and disrespect and are the target of comic relief on stage. If the benefits of soluble fiber don't outweigh your concern over the gas produced, you will need to limit your fiber intake to

the insoluble fibers.

2. Q: I want a fiber that will be best for my diverticulosis and help to prevent episodes of diverticulitis.
A: The medical literature will show that insoluble fibers are the best solution for this request, though some doctors will beg to differ based upon how long ago they were trained. Start with low doses of wheat fiber (like All Bran cereal) and slowly work your way up to a minimum of either 14 grams for every 1000 calories consumed or 40 gms/day. The literature also shows there is no need to avoid nuts and seeds as many practicing physicians still suggest. However, like anything else in medicine, listen to your body. If popcorn or flaxseed cause you abdominal discomfort, then you should avoid them.

   If, for whatever reason, there is a soluble fiber that you prefer over an insoluble one, both soluble and insoluble fibers will help to alleviate constipation and the consequent high colonic pressures required to evacuate any fecal contents. Be sure to drink adequate fluids and avoid stimulant laxatives.

For active cases of diverticulitis, it *is* normal protocol to aid the healing bowel by placing it "at rest" with low residue (fiber) diets until healing is fully achieved. In addition, your doctor may place you on antibiotics—or even recommend surgery for severe or refractory disease.

3. Q: I want a fiber to prevent me from ever developing diverticulosis.

A: Although there are no guarantees for anything in life, for someone with no history of diverticulosis and who presumably has a normal and healthy bowel, a combination of both soluble and insoluble fibers appears to be a prudent approach. I think nature proves the best teacher by providing an equal portion of each in natural oatmeal or a 2:1 ratio (of soluble to insoluble fiber) with psyllium. Hence, one reasonable option is to consume relatively equal weights of wheat fiber and a soluble fiber throughout the day. Under ideal circumstances (which I recognize are not always practical), I would recommend consuming the insoluble and soluble fibers distributed equally throughout the day and with each meal. There is no great value to consuming any fiber outside of mealtime (although I suspect some unusual situations may exist). Psyllium powder, especially for travelers or for eating at the workplace, offers the convenience of being able to carry it in a small container to supplement with your meals.

4. Q: I want a fiber that will help me with my elevated cholesterol.
A: The University of Maryland Medical Center website recommends the following:

Soluble fibers, such as those in

psyllium husk (which contains both soluble and insoluble fiber), guar gum, flax seed, and oat bran, can help lower cholesterol when added to a low saturated fat, low cholesterol diet. Clinical studies show that psyllium, in particular, is effective in lowering total cholesterol levels as well as LDL (or "bad") cholesterol levels.[43]

Certainly, the studies cited in **Chapter 2** also support this added benefit of the soluble fibers.

5. Q: I want a fiber that will help my irritable bowel disease.
A: Studies indicate that most soluble fibers will aid with this problem.

6. Q: I want a fiber that will help my inflammatory bowel disease (IBD).
A: Patients with these problematic diseases are often benefited by a fermentable soluble fiber such as psyllium. IBD patients should consult with their physicians for advice on

their particular need.

7. Q: I want a fiber that will not constipate me.

A: Probably any fiber has the potential for causing constipation when adequate liquids are not simultaneously consumed—though the soluble fibers pose the greatest risk for this hazard. As long as you take in adequate fluids, neither type of fiber should cause a problem with constipation.

If you have a history of chronic constipation however, the insoluble fibers should be your first choice.

8. Q: I want a fiber that will not give me diarrhea.

A: Insoluble fibers pose the greatest risk for loose bowel movements, especially when the unaccustomed bowel is suddenly introduced to them. The unaccustomed bowel should be introduced to any fiber at low volumes and with gradual increases.

Soluble fibers, on the other hand,

are often used to treat conditions associated with diarrhea and represent the fibers of choice for these conditions. You will still need to ingest sufficient liquids, however, despite having diarrhea.

9. Q: I want a fiber that won't react with the medications I take.
A: Any fiber has this unfortunate potential, and you will need to check with your physician for advice on this topic. Most physicians will recommend that any oral medications be taken at least 1 hour *before* or 2 - 4 hours *after* taking any fiber product.[44]

10. Q: I want a fiber with no side effects.
A: Despite the relative safety of most fibers, recommendations on fiber supplementation will vary depending upon your particular health condition. You should check with your physician for advice on this topic.

11. Q: Will fiber supplementation help

me to lose weight?

A: A feeling of satiety or fullness is one of the best "side effects" to taking dietary fiber. Additionally, recent studies support the production of various agents which suppress hunger through the central nervous system. If your physician approves of you taking fiber with your meals, I recommend that you time your fiber consumption for the first half of your meal, drink the necessary additional fluids, and eat at a slow pace. The idea is to give the fiber the necessary time to fully expand within the confines of your stomach so as to induce early satiety and help you to reduce your immediate intake of calories. For added security against any concern regarding diminished nutrient (e.g., vitamin) absorption, you might consider simply taking a daily multiple vitamin with your largest meal.

Since no text can be all-inclusive or comprehensive, this short text is no exception. Hopefully, however, this book has piqued enough of an interest in the human alimentary system to stimulate beneficial changes in your diet and other health practices.

The cultures of our developing countries have inadvertently done much to reduce and alter the healthy lifestyles to which our bowels have so successfully evolved.

Fiber, for one, is again proving that what once was old is now new.

Index

Endnotes:

[1] Shinta Cho. *The Gas We Pass*. Brooklyn, New York: Kane/Miller Book Publishers, 1994.

[2] Higgins, P. D., Johanson, J. F. "Epidemiology of constipation in North America: a systemic Review." *Am J Gastroenterol*. 2004 Apr; 99 (4): 750-9. <http://www.ncbi.nlm.nih.gov/m/pubmed/150899 11> Retrieved 14 June 2013.

[3] Rome III Diagnostic Criteria for Functional Gastrointestinal   Disorders <http://www.romecriteria.org/assets/pdf/19_Rom eIII_apA_885-898.pdf> Retrieved 11 March 2015.

[4] Diverticulitis occurs in approximately 10–25% of people with diverticulosis.

[5] This daily recommendation of fiber is for the prevention of coronary disease.

[6] Institute of Medicine. "Dietary Reference Intakes for Energy, Carbohydrate, Fiber, Fat, Fatty Acids, Cholesterol, Protein, and Amino Acids." Washington, DC: The National Academies Press. 2005. <http://books.nap.edu/openbook.php?isbn=03090 85373> Retrieved 19 March 2013.

[7] Burkitt, Denis. *Don't forget fibre in your diet: to help avoid many of our commonest diseases*. London: Martin Dunitz Ltd., 1979.

[8] The World Health Organization defines diarrhea as "the passage of 3 or more loose or liquid stools per day, or more frequently than is normal for the individual"[<http://www.who.int/topics/diarrhoea /en/> (2015)] .

[9]   A   medically-recognized   syndrome "characterized   by   chronic   abdominal   pain, discomfort,   bloating,   and   alteration   of   bowel habits.   Diarrhea   or   constipation   may predominate, or they may alternate (classified as IBS-D,   IBS-C,   or   IBS-A,   respectively)" [<http://en.wikipedia.org/wiki/Irritable_bowel_sy ndrome> (5 March 2015)].

[10]   Whiteman,   Honor.   "How   a   fiber-rich   diet protects   against   obesity   and   diabetes." <http://www.medicalnewstoday.com/articles/271 220.php>   (15   January   2014)   Retrieved   20 February 2015.

[11]   Emspak,   Jesse.   "Why   High-Fiber   Diets   May Help   Weight   Loss." <http://www.livescience.com/45225-why-fiber- helps-weight-loss.html>   (29   April   2014) Retrieved 20 February 2015.

[12]   Owens,   Brian.   "Dietary   fibre   acts   on   brain   to suppress   appetite." <http://www.nature.com/news/dietary-fibre-acts- on-brain-to-suppress-appetite.htm>   (29   April 2014) Retrieved 20 February 2015.

[13] A similar product, Post's 100% Bran, is no longer available.

[14] Research has demonstrated that one observable, normal change following the added intake of fiber is an increase in the size of the cecum (also caecum) or proximal colon.

[15] Similar stories may be recited regarding the history of wine, chocolate, eggs, and even the once-advocated clean environment for growing infants.

[16] Coffee is known to contain a protein moiety responsible for elevating the low-density lipoprotein (LDL) component of cholesterol. This constituent is removed when coffee passes through the commonly sold paper filters found in grocery stores.

[17] Weisberger L, Jamieson B. "Clinical inquiries: How can you help prevent a recurrence of diverticulitis?" *J Fam Pract.* July 2009. 58(7): 381-2.

[18] Digestive Health Center Nutrition Services. "Low Fiber Diet for Diverticulitis." Stanford Hospital and Clinics. July 2007.

[19] University of Maryland Medical Center (UMMC). "Diverticular Disease." Baltimore, MD: UMMC. 2011. <http://www.umm.edu/altmed/articles/diverticular-disease-000051.htm> Retrieved 23 March 2013.

[20] UCSF. "Diverticular Disease and Diet." <http://www.ucsfhealth.org/education/diverticular_disease_and_diet/> Retrieved 24 March 2013.

[21] NIH Publication No. 08–1163. "Diverticulosis and Diverticulitis." July 2008. http://digestive.niddk.nih.gov/ddiseases/pubs/diverticulosis/ Retrieved 24 March 2013.

[22] Cleveland Clinic Foundation. "Diverticular Disease." Cleveland, OH: Cleveland Clinic Foundation. 10 September 2012. <http://my.clevelandclinic.org/disorders/diverticulosis/diverticulitis/hic_diverticular_disease.aspx> Retrieved 24 March 2013.

[23] Institute of Medicine. "Dietary Reference Intakes for Energy, Carbohydrate, Fiber, Fat, Fatty Acids, Cholesterol, Protein, and Amino Acids." Washington, DC: The National Academies Press. 2005. <http://books.nap.edu/openbook.php?isbn=0309085373> Retrieved 19 March 2013.

[24] University of Maryland Medical Center (UMMC). "Fiber." Baltimore, MD: UMMC. 2011. http://www.umm.edu/altmed/articles/fiber-000303.htm. Retrieved 29 March 2013.

[25] Spence, J. David; Huff, Murray W.; Heidenheim, Paul; Viswanatha, Anne; Munoz, Claudio; Lindsay, Robert; Wolfe, Bernard; and Mills, Donald. "Combination Therapy with

Colestipol and Psyllium Mucilloid in Patients with Hyperlipidemia." *Annals of Internal Medicine.* 1995 1 Oct. 123 (7): 493-499.

[26] Dam, B. P.; O'Connell, N. C.; Jerdack, G. R.; Stinson, B. A.; Sptrhell, K. D. R. "Additive hypocholesterolemic effect of psyllium and cholestyramine in the hamster influence on fecal sterol and bile acid profiles." *J Lipid Res.* 1997 Mar; 38(3): 491-502.
<http://www.jlr.org/cgi/issue_pdf/toc_pdf/38/3.pdf>

[27] Monnier, L., Phma, T. C., Aguirre, L., Orsetti, A., Mirouze. "Influence of Indigestible Fibers on Glucose Tolerance." J. *Diabetes Care J.* March-April 1978: 83-88.
<http://care.diabetesjournals.org/content/1/2/83.full.pdf> Retrieved 2 June 2013.

[28] University of Maryland Medical Center (UMMC). "Hypoglycemia." Baltimore, MD: UMMC. 2011.
<http://www.umm.edu/altmed/articles/hypoglycemia-000090.htm> Retrieved 29 March 2013.

[29] Although this text is not formally a weight-loss guide, I would like to cite one incentive that is often overlooked. Consider, if you are only 25 pounds overweight, it is the equivalent of carrying three 1-gallon containers of water on your person 24 hours a day!

[30] Wikipedia.org. "Psyllium seed husks."

<http://en.wikipedia.org/wiki/Psyllium_seed_hus ks> (24 February 2013). Retrieved 24 March 2013.

[31] Institute of Medicine. "Dietary Reference Intakes for Energy, Carbohydrate, Fiber, Fat, Fatty Acids, Cholesterol, Protein, and Amino Acids." Washington, DC: The National Academies Press. 2005. <http://books.nap.edu/openbook.php?isbn=03090 85373> Retrieved 19 March 2013.

[32] Horowitz, Bruce. "Kellogg adds fiber, hoping to bowl cereal consumers over." *USA Today*. 2009 4 June; Section 3B.

[33] www.WebMD.com. "Natural Colon Cleansing: Is It Necessary?" <http://www.webmd.com/balance/guide/natural-colon-cleansing-is-it-necessary?page=3> Retrieved 10 April 2013

[34] www.WebMD.com. "Natural Colon Cleansing: Is It Necessary?" <http://www.webmd.com/balance/guide/natural-colon-cleansing-is-it-necessary?page=3> Retrieved 10 April 2013

[35] www.WebMD.com. "Natural Colon Cleansing: Is It Necessary?" <http://www.webmd.com/balance/guide/natural-colon-cleansing-is-it-necessary?page=2> Retrieved 10 April 2013

[36] www.WebMD.com. "Natural Colon Cleansing: Is It Necessary?" <http://www.webmd.com/balance/guide/natural-colon-cleansing-is-it-necessary?page=2> Retrieved 10 April 2013

[37] Aroniadis, Olga C., Brandt, Lawrence J. *Curr. Opin. Gastroenterol.* 2013: 29 (1): 79-84. <www.medscape.com/viewarticle/776501_9> Retrieved 5 June 2013.

[38] Behar, J., Hitchings, M., Smyth, R. D. "Calcium stimulation of gastrin and gastric acid secretion: effect of small doses of calcium carbonate" *Gut*, 1977, 18, 442-448. <http://www.ncbi.nlm.nih.gov/pmc/articles/PMC 1411522/pdf/gut00475-0028.pdf> Retrieved 29 May 2013

[39] Hardman, Joel G., Gilman, Alfred Goodman, Limbird, Lee E. *Goodman and Gilman's THE PHARMACOLOGIC BASIS OF THERAPEUTICS*. USA: The McGraw-Hill Companies, Inc., 1996, pp. 910-12.

[40] Wikipedia.org. "Simethicone." <http://en.wikipedia.org/wiki/simethicone> (25 May 2013). Retrieved 1 June 2013.

[41] Wikipedia.org. "Proton-pump inhibitor." <http://en.wikipedia.org/wiki/Proton-pump_inhibitor> (29 May 2013). Retrieved 31 May 2013.

[42] Bockus, M.D., Henry, et.al.. *Gastroenterology*. Philadelphia: W. B. Saunders, 1964, p. 754

[43]University of Maryland Medical Center (UMMC). "Fiber." Baltimore, MD: UMMC. 2011. <http://www.umm.edu/altmed/articles/fiber-000303.htm> Retrieved 29 March 2013.

[44] University of Maryland Medical Center (UMMC). "Fiber." Baltimore, MD: UMMC. 2011. <http://www.umm.edu/altmed/articles/fiber-000303.htm> Retrieved 29 March 2013.